Chronic Fatigue Syndrome: Living Your Life without the Limits of CFS

KARA AIMER

CONTENTS

INTRODUCTION

I want to personally thank you for picking up the book, Chronic Fatigue Syndrome. This book contains proven steps and strategies to get your life back on track and to go above and beyond the limits of this somewhat common, yet unfortunate and debilitating condition. Chronic fatigue syndrome (CFS) is a health disorder in which patients showcase prolonged fatigue (which can last for months or even years) as the primary symptom, among other minor symptoms. Irrespective of the amount or quality of the rest taken, the patient is not relieved of the fatigue. There has been no medical condition that has been proven through research to clearly explain this disorder. However, it is apparent that increased mental and physical activity worsens the symptoms of the disorder. Although the real cause of this disorder is not yet scientifically proven through research, theories that try to explain their origin range from psychological distress and time zones to genetics and viral infections, among others. It cannot be diagnosed by a single test, but in order to rule out other medical conditions that showcase symptoms that are similar, many other medical examinations must be carried out by a doctor or team of physicians. Stress, age, gender, depression, and psychological factors are the main risk factors for developing this disorder.

Chronic fatigue syndrome is a common disorder in our modern society, according to a particular study carried out in the recent past. According to the study, whose respondents ages ranged from 20 years old to 50 years old, three in every 1,000 Americans suffer from this disorder. This clearly shows how common Chronic Fatigue Syndrome is, globally and nationally. It is not easy living a healthy lifestyle in the modern world, with technology having made almost everything too simple and reachable with just a click of the mouse. Because of our lack of movement and thinking for ourselves, we have seen many diseases gain traction, with some of them having no cure at all while others can be taken care of through lifestyle changes or medication. It takes a significant amount of effort to live actively and healthily through self-discipline, patience, and enthusiasm. This does not mean that it is impossible for someone to live life abundantly without any kind of limitation brought about by this illness. It just takes an extra amount of energy and self-drive, to reach one's target.

This book explains the different theories of causes, symptoms, and diagnoses of this chronic disorder. Although CFS has no cure, this book discusses the various treatments that are used to reduce or eliminate its range of symptoms. Supplements and diets of CFS will be thoroughly explained in the book. There are many dietary supplements that can be administered to CFS patients and approved exercises or activities that they are allowed to perform as part of their treatment. When it comes to this disorder of chronic fatigue, there are so many do's and don'ts that you must know as well. Management of stress is inevitable, and this book clearly explains what it takes to keep this monster at bay, as a way of living life to the fullest and feeling better while doing it. Whether you are struggling with this condition, looking for information on how to live a healthy life without this menace, or just wanting to learn something new about CFS, this book will be very helpful to you and those you love. Find out for yourself how you can live a life without the limits of CFS in this fast-paced life. Thanks again for picking up this book, I hope you enjoy it!

Also, don't forget to grab your FREE Bonuses via the link at the end!

A quick disclaimer: This book is not intended to suggest or replace medical advice. The information contained in this work is intended as general information only. The information presented is not intended to diagnose, treat or cure any health issues or take the place of professional medical care. For persistent health issues or further questions, please consult your health care provider.

Now, let's get to it!

THEORIES OF CAUSES AND SYMPTOMS AND DIAGNOSES

There are many theories that try to explain the causes, symptoms, and diagnoses of Chronic Fatigue Syndrome. There is no single cause of CFS that has been proven through research to be the root cause of all its cases or incidences; neither brain scans nor blood tests can be used for the definite diagnosis of this medical disorder. According to various experts in this field, there are many factors that converge to cause CFS, such as genetics, abnormalities in the brain, a hyper-reactive immune system, infectious or viral agents, as well as emotional or psychiatric disorders. As an example, before the patient is diagnosed with CFS, they report emotional events similar to those resulting from depression or severe to moderate physical ailments like viral infections that are chronic.

According to the theories by other experts, in this arena, CFS is triggered when a certain event or combination of events interact with particular genetic or neurologic abnormalities. However, the cause of prominent symptoms such as fatigue in a patient with CFS, in their sequential order of occurrence, is still a mystery. Equally puzzling is the brain: experts pinpoint any particular problem in the nervous or the brain system to be the cause of this medical disorder. Five of the most popular theories that try to explain the causes of this disorder are discussed below.

CFS can be linked to genes that control stressful events such as injury and response to trauma. These genes are found in the sympathetic nervous system and the hypothalamic-pituitary axis of the adrenal gland. However, it is not clear how these genetic factors affect the symptoms of CFS. Various research studies have indicated changes in the cell communication, immune function, and cell energy transfer genes in patients with this disorder. Although no clear pattern has been determined through these studies, most of the genes identified by researchers are associated with the functions of the immune system, diseases of the blood and infections.

Abnormalities in Hormones and the Central Nervous System

The brain regulates certain kinds of chemicals in the body referred to as the hypothalamus-pituitary-adrenal (HPA) axis. According to this theory, the abnormal levels of this chemical cause chronic fatigue syndrome. Response to stress, sleep, and depression, are some body functions controlled by the central nervous system. Changes in critical neurotransmitters, such low levels of dopamine and high levels of serotonin are said to bring about Chronic Fatigue Syndrome. Low levels of cortisol, a stress hormone, have been determined to bring about a weaker or impaired response to physical or psychological stress like exercises and infections, respectively. Although some patients showed improvement when administered cortisol supplements, others did not.

Disturbance of the circadian rhythms that cause the sleep-wake cycle disorder is also said to cause CFS. Found in the HPA axis, this is a nerve cluster that is controlled by the circadian clock. Repeated disturbance of sleep occurs when the rhythms are not reset as expected for proper functioning of the body. Certain medications taken by some CFS patients were found to work and thus help improve their disorders. No study has proven that indeed these alterations in certain body chemicals cause CFS, however.

Infections

According to many researchers, there is a possibility of certain CFS symptoms being caused by viral infections because they are similar to those of certain viral ailments. However, not all patients with this medical disorder showcase similar symptoms to that of an infection, nor do they show similar symptoms to each other. Despite controversies surrounding the theory that viruses may cause CFS, this disorder can be either viral or non-viral. Organisms that bring about Lyme disease, measles, Candida or yeast infection, Epstein-Barr herpes virus type 6 (HHV-6), Coxsackie B, parvovirus, human T cell lymph tropic virus (HTLV). Even cytomegalovirus are said to increase the levels of antibodies in CFS patients. Starting as a flue, about 80% of this disorder are said to begin as such. However, unlike infections, no evidence exists to prove that intimate sexual or casual contact such as coughing and hand shaking, spread this disorder from one person to another.

According to the CDC, chronic fatigue syndrome is not contagious and mainly takes place sporadically, but this has been proven otherwise in the US where cluster outbreaks in the workplaces, households, and communities have been reported.

Abnormalities in the Immune System

Commonly known as the chronic fatigue immune dysfunction syndrome, several studies have found abnormalities in the immune system. With a lack of consistency to categorize CFS as an immune system disorder, some elements are said to be under-reactive while others over-reactive. Most CFS patients are said to be allergic to pollens, foods and metals like mercury and nickel. According to one theory, viral infections are considered allergens that can trigger abnormalities in the immune system, and thus causing chronic fatigue syndrome. Despite this fact, those who are allergic do not have CFS. Autoimmune disease risk profiles resemble those of CFS. However, in patients with the fatigue syndrome that is chronic, research has failed to provide consistent results to show the presence of auto-antibodies; these kinds of antibodies attack body tissues. Therefore, auto-immunity is unlikely to be the cause of this syndrome in most people.

Low Blood Pressure

Patients with CFS have been proven, by research, to showcase symptoms of NMH (Naturally Mediated Hypotension). When a patient with NMH stands up, their blood pressure drops instantly with effects such as nausea, lightheadedness, and fainting. Despite this fact, no evidence exists to prove that CFS patients have a high risk of having NMH.

Psychological Factors

CFS is related to personality, emotional, and social factors. However, there is no proper understanding of the relationship between emotional and physical factors that are said to be very complex. Furthermore, no research has found evidence to show that there is a consistent relationship between CFS and either personality or emotional disorders. Therefore, it is not likely that psychological factors can be an important cause of chronic fatigue syndrome. However, there is a chance that they play a role in a person's likelihood of having this chronic disorder. Actually, it is this disorder that enhances social and emotional dysfunction in many patients.

TREATMENT OF CFS SYMPTOMS

Chronic fatigue syndrome has no cure and treatment is only aimed at relieving the patient of the symptoms. Some symptoms of this disorder comprise of fatigue, sore throat, muscle pains, poor quality of sleep, and insomnia, tender lymph nodes, impairment in concentration or memory, severe headaches, joint pains without swelling or redness, low energy, feelings of worthlessness or guilt, suicidal thoughts, depression and anxiety, significant loss and gain in weight, loss of interest, recklessness and lack of concentration or decision-making. Treatment can improve the condition of CFS patients, such as disorders related to psychology and depression. A combination of the following therapies, techniques, and medications, are used in the treatment of CFS.

Cognitive Behavioral Therapy (CBT)

CBT is a treatment that alters how a CFS patient behaves and thinks; it is used in the treatment of various health conditions. It does not just aim to reduce the symptoms of chronic fatigue syndrome, but also distress that is related to it. The cycle of interconnected negative emotions, thoughts, actions and physical sensations as well as problems that overwhelm a patient are broken down into smaller bits, using this treatment. The therapy uses a one-on-one approach to offer treatment and a program is designed by an experienced therapist to suit the specific patient's needs because what might work for a particular patient might not work for another.

Diagnosis acceptance, challenging of negative thoughts that worsen symptoms and development of the patient's self-control over the symptoms might encompass the programs designed for patients under CBT. In addition to mental conditions, CBT is also used in the treatment of rheumatoid arthritis and cancer. Therefore, chronic fatigue syndrome is not a mental condition.

Graded Exercise Therapy

This is a program for structured training aimed at increasing the duration of physical activities in patients, gradually. Aerobic exercises such as walking and swimming that increase heart rate are included in a GET program. Depending on the patient's physical ability, the exercises included in their programs are picked accordingly. Just like CBT, it is offered as a one-on-one approach by an expert with experience handling CFS cases. Exercise intensity and duration of physical activity is gradually increased with time as the patient adjusts to their program. All therapy sessions must be conducted within the scope of the program. Goals must also be set by both the therapist and the patient; they must be achieved in the long run even if it takes weeks, months or years.

Management of Activity

Activity management is an essential component of a CFS treatment program, and it entails goal setting and gradual increment of the level of activity. Keeping a diary can help the patient establish a baseline from where they can tell if they are ready for longer periods of activity.

Medication

Although there is no medication that can cure this disorder, they are used to reduce CFS symptoms. Medication mainly used to reduce fatigue, discomfort, pain, fever, anxiety and depression. Painkillers can be used to reduce pain in patients with this disorder; however, strong ones should not be taken by patients for a long time. There are pain management clinics, like in the UK, which specialize in the management of chronic pains. Antidepressants such as Amitriptyline can be prescribed to CFS patients who have problems falling asleep; it is not recommended for those with heart problems, though. Blurred vision, dryness of the mouth, drowsiness and dizziness are some side effects of using this drug. Anti-emetic is for patients with severe nausea.

Lifestyle/Self-Help Techniques
Here are some other methods of treating chronic fatigue syndrome:

- Breathing and relaxation techniques
- Pacing (balancing of rest and activity periods)

- Taking frequent breaks between activities
- Being optimistic about eventually getting cured
- Sleep and stress management techniques
- Living a healthy lifestyle
- Avoiding foods the patient is sensitive to
- Hypnosis
- Massage therapies
- Biofeedback
- Meditation
- Yoga
- Avoidance of caffeine, alcohol, sweeteners and sugar

Aromatherapy, herbal, and home remedies and alternative medicine such as Ayurvedic medicine are also used in treating chronic fatigue syndrome. These treatments can help avoid relapses if used well. It takes time to overcome CFS, but with patience and discipline to stick to a treatment program, a patient can completely recover, in the long run.

NATURAL TREATMENTS FOR CFS

Although alternative medicine use is quite prevalent among patients and families who suffer from chronic fatigue syndrome, one must keep in mind that there is very little scientific support for the claim that any form of alternative medicine can treat chronic fatigue syndrome. Part of that is just because it has not actually been studied extensively by mainstream scientists or top universities. However, there are a few that people have reported work well and helped them. You may have to try a few of these before you find something that works for you and your particular symptoms.

Ginseng

Ginseng is a herb that has been used in Asia for centuries to increase energy and combat fatigue, but you may know it better as the thing that is in excellent green teas. A survey of 155 people who suffer from CFS or other forms of constant fatigue done by researchers at the University of Iowa found that ginseng was considered one of the most helpful treatment options given to them. Fifty-six percent of people who used ginseng rating it as effective in helping the symptoms of their chronic fatigue.

Another study found that a particular type of ginseng, Panax ginseng, significantly enhanced cellular immune function by peripheral mononuclear cells. These blood cells are a critical component of the immune system as they fight infection in people with chronic fatigue syndrome or acquired immunodeficiency syndrome (AIDS).

However, in another study done by a top tier university, a double-blinded, placebo-controlled study involving 96 people with persistent fatigue found that another type of ginseng, Siberian ginseng, was no better than placebo at reducing fatigue.

Nicotinamide Adenine Dinucleotide (NADH)

Nicotinamide Adenine Dinucleotide (NADH) is a naturally occurring molecule formed from vitamin B3 (niacin) that plays an essential role in cellular energy production. Previously, it had been used in studies for cancer, AIDS, and muscle repairs. Now, it is being tested on chronic fatigue patients. Stay tuned for the results – though they look to be very, very promising.

L-Carnitine

Carnitine, found in nearly all body cells, is responsible for transporting long-chain fatty acids into mitochondria, the energy-producing centers of cells. It allows these fatty acids to be converted into energy, mainly making this the source of fuel for our bodies – it keeps us moving – something those who suffer from CFS have trouble doing.

Some studies have found that carnitine levels in the body are decreased in people with chronic fatigue syndrome and it has been linked to muscle fatigue and pain and impaired exercise tolerance. However, other studies haven't found an association between carnitine deficiency and symptoms of chronic fatigue syndrome.

One study examined the use of L-carnitine in 30 people with chronic fatigue syndrome. After 8 weeks of treatment, there was statistically significant clinical improvement in 12 of the 18 parameters, with the greatest improvement occurring after 4 weeks of treatment. Some participants reported that they were sick. There was no placebo group in this study and it wasn't blinded, so more clinical trials are needed.

Coenzyme Q10

Coenzyme Q10 (Co Q10) is a compound found naturally in the mitochondria, the energy-producing center of our cells. Co Q10 is involved in the production of ATP, the primary energy source of body cells. Co Q10 is also an antioxidant. A survey of 155 people with persistent fatigue found that the percentage of users who found a treatment helpful was greatest for Co Q10 (69% of 13 people).

Dehydroepiandrosterone (DHEA)

DHEA is a hormone secreted by the adrenal glands and in smaller amounts by the ovaries and testes. DHEA can be converted in the body to other steroid hormones, such as estrogen and testosterone. It is also involved in memory, mood, and sleep. Levels of DHEA in the body peak when a person is in his or her mid-20s and then slowly decline with age.

Studies have shown that DHEA levels are slightly abnormal to very abnormal in people with chronic fatigue syndrome. DHEA is not recommended unless lab tests indicate there is a deficiency. Treatment should be closely supervised by a qualified health practitioner. Little is known about the long-term safety of DHEA.

Because DHEA is converted to estrogen and testosterone, people with estrogen- and testosterone-related conditions, such as breast, ovarian, prostate, and testicular cancer should avoid DHEA or at least talk to their doctor and weigh the pros and cons. Adverse effects of DHEA include high blood pressure, lowered HDL ("good") cholesterol, and liver toxicity. DHEA can increase testosterone in women and result in male pattern baldness, weight gain, acne, deepening of the voice, and other signs of masculinization.

DIET/SUPPLEMENTS FOR CFS

Nutrition should also be used as a therapy in the management and treatment of chronic fatigue syndrome. It does not just boost the immune system as part of health improvement, but also eliminates dietary elements that might play a role in aggravating the symptoms of this disorder. A perfect diet for CFS patients should incorporate whole foods that are not refined as these will be high in fiber and complex carbohydrates but low in fats, sugar, and animal proteins. Garlic and astragal roots have anti-bacterial properties, therefore, can fight bacteria, fungi, and viruses; therefore, should be included in the patient's diet. Caffeine has an adverse effect on the adrenaline, therefore, should be avoided entirely. An elimination diet should be used to determine the foods that the patient is allergic to by avoiding the foods they are sensitive to for about 2 weeks before reintroducing them one by one.

In order to support the adrenal glands and the immune system, patients can be administered diet supplements such as beta-carotene, vitamin C, zinc, adrenal extracts, sodium, magnesium mixed with malic acid and vitamin B5 or pantothenic acid. Yeast found in the body known as Candida multiplies a lot with prolonged use of antibiotics. Yeast overgrowth can be managed by eating a diet rich in fruits and vegetables rich in antioxidant, omega-3 fatty acids found in certain oils and fish, honey, corn syrup and dairy products that contain lactose. All foods that are cooked, prepared, baked or fermented with yeast must be avoided. Extracts of grapefruit seeds and Caprylic acid should also be included in the diet. A good example of a nutritional prescription for this disorder can encompass adrenal extract tablets, a supplement that contains many vitamins and minerals, as well as malic acid and magnesium supplements.

Water is also an essential dietary element. Therefore, patients should be sure to drink enough water every day. If possible, up to a maximum of 8 liters is recommended. Other supplements include vitamins B-complex and 100, antioxidants, 500mg of Eleuthero three times in a day and coenzyme Q10 that can be taken on a daily basis of 60-120 mg.

ACTIVITY/EXERCISE FOR CFS TREATMENT AND MANAGEMENT

Activities or exercises done on a regular basis can help manage chronic fatigue syndrome and reduce the severe effects of its symptoms. Research shows that moderate exercise can decrease distress, fatigue and symptoms as well as pains related to CFS. Moreover, it improves aerobic fitness, physical functions and perceptions of health. According to other studies, the ability to perform activities on a daily basis and CFS symptoms can be significantly improved by engaging in exercises of moderate intensity such as pool exercises and walking. The study correspondents reported less muscle pain and fewer joint pains. No matter how difficult or painful it might be to begin exercising or engaging in light activity, the pain cycle must be broken by the patient to start feeling better and return to a normal life.

Benefits of Activity/Exercise

For patients struggling with CFS, there are numerous health benefits that result from participating in physical activities or exercises. These benefits include:

- Enhanced performance in recreational activities and work
- Decreased anxiety, stress and depression
- Increased energy
- Decreased blood pressure and heart rate during rests
- Improved sense of well-being
- Improved sleep
- Improved profile of cholesterol

- Decreased fatigue and pain
- Decreased risk of getting a stroke or a heart disease
- Decreased muscle and joint pains
- Improved blood sugar level control
- Enhanced fat burning ability
- Enhanced physical fitness
- Improved heart efficiency
- Decreased loss of aerobic fitness and strength of the muscles

Getting Started with a Customized Exercise Program

Activities to be performed on a daily basis are increased gradually from the first day of beginning an exercise program. As an example, a person with this disorder should take advantage of every possible opportunity of getting physically active. Take some extra walks, use stairs instead of elevators, and do more housing chores. Limit sitting around and use computers or watch TV less often. It is only a doctor who can determine whether a patient is ready for an exercise program or not. Exercise programs should begin slowly and as the body adjusts to the physical activities, intensity and duration should be gradually increased. Symptoms can be aggravated if a patient starts to exercise intensively before the body is used to the new physical activities. Having fatigue and feeling sore should be expected as is normal. Activities that worsen symptoms or make one feel more tired should be avoided.

Types of Exercises and Fitness programs Recommended for CFS

Aerobic and stretching exercises are highly recommended for treating and managing CFS. Swimming, walking, water aerobics, rowing a machine and riding a stationary bike are some excellent aerobic exercises that can be adopted by CFS patients to increase heart rate and blood flow to all parts of the body. In addition to stretching exercises, breathing techniques and yoga also improve the supply of nutrients and blood to the joints and thus leading to increased coordination, reduction in stress on the muscles, decreased injury risks and improved balance. Conditioning and strengthening exercises are also recommended. On the first day, patients can exercise for as little as 5 minutes and 1 to 2 times per week. This should be increased slowly over time until the patient can exercise for 30 minutes per day, 3 days per week.

The intensity of the exercise should only be increased once the patient suffering from chronic fatigue syndrome is comfortable with working out for 30 minutes continuously in a day. Strength training can then be introduced into the exercise program. Training level and intensity should always be consistent, irrespective of how good or bad the patient feels in any given day. It is important to listen to one's own body and only increase intensity when the body is ready to take that next step. Any abnormal pain should mean that the patient is over doing it, hence must stop and have a rest.

CFS patients also benefit from improved health as a result of exercising. They say that it is better late than never. Therefore, patients should take a step now and make the effort needed to begin exercising as part of living an active and healthy lifestyle in addition to relieving the pain and fatigue associated with this disorder.

ORGANIZING YOUR HOME AND CAR

When you have CFS, organizing your daily life can make a huge change when it comes to how you cope and get around. CFS can make it nearly impossible to complete tasks and keep an orderly lifestyle. However, there are some tips and trick that you can learn when it comes to keeping each accessible, orderly, and safe for you and your entire family.

The Home

People with chronic illness often have problems with housecleaning and the control of the clutter they have sitting around in all environments. Once a home reaches a certain stage of disarray, it can seem hopeless to people who are entirely healthy. For CFS, is can be extremely detrimental not only to your body, but also to your mind and self-esteem. Living this way contributes to emotional distress and social isolation, as people feel embarrassed about having guests, making plans, or even having romantic conquests.

Once you are able to address these issues, you will feel better about yourself, your home, and your life, in general.

Common Problems

Your ability to do housework like cleaning and organizing may gradually decrease over the years if you don't have a firm grasp on it or if your health declines. You can always try to get help from your family, set up a schedule so everyone would do some of the chores around the house, or even hiring someone out. It's all time (and energy) consuming which is something that you don't need.

You probably won't get much cooperation, and even with that, clutter might still keep building up and you will face the same problems again and again.

Common Answers

There is really one simple answer to making your home a clean, organized, and welcoming place when you don't have the energy to do so. Surely, there are articles about it in housekeeping magazines and such that tell you how to stay clean and orderly forever, but you have to have the energy to even get to that point. Rather, it may take a combination of a lot of things to go from chaos to comfort – including you pushing your mind and body.

The first idea is to just live a life that is better suited for CFS sufferers. Those might be small little things that will give you the strength to tackle your home room by room. You should rest before you get tired, take it easy, and focus only on the things that really matter. It won't matter if that room you never use doesn't get dusted or vacuumed this week. Try to meditate twice daily, once before and once after you clean, and lie down to rest for fifteen minutes with your eyes closed once or twice a day, especially if you are particularly stressed out.

You could also work out better systems for dealing with disarray, dirt, and clutter. For example, you could sort the mail as soon as it arrives, instead of letting it pile up. Throw away or recycle what you do not want, put the bills in a safe place or pay them right away if you can. Put the mail you wish to look over later in some bins placed on shelves by your chair. Make sure the other members of your home know about their own mail, and then move on. Don't stockpile things you don't want. If it makes it easier, keep a shredder by your desk for easy removal.

The biggest thing is that you don't try to reform everything at once, but rather you should change things gradually. For example, you might notice that your bathroom vanity top was so filled with bottles, jars, and other things that you, your family, and guests could barely use the sink. Go ahead and clear it off. Take away the things that you don't use on a daily basis, throw away things that are so old they might be science experiments, and try to focus on organizing what you absolutely need to have on the top of your vanity. You can do this slowly, even if you just organize while you are using the bathroom for something. Once you are done there, move on to somewhere else in the room.

When you have to do a big project like cleaning a closet or reorganizing the garage, do not try to get it done in one day. Instead, you should assign yourself one shelf or one rack of clothes to go through on a particular day. Sometimes it will work best if you only tell yourself to do 15 minutes worth of work and stop at the end of that time. The next day or even later on in that day, you can do another 15 minutes until eventually the whole closet will be clean and organized.

Also, you should start to congratulate yourself for your efforts and for what you have accomplished, even if you didn't do as much as a healthy person would do. You will come to see that, like other chronically ill people, you are always making a huge effort, so you always have something for which you can congratulate yourself. And focusing on what you have done is much better for you psychologically than blaming yourself for what was yet undone.

With your new understanding of progress through small, actionable steps, you will have success by involving your family by asking them to use a similar strategy. If everyone does just 15 minutes of work twice a day, you might actually be accomplishing more than ever.

It might take you several years to move from the chaos you currently have a neat and organized home. This is because you aren't just cleaning up, you are re-training yourself in your approach to housework. You will have setbacks: weeks where you don't feel like doing anything and the clutter builds up. Just start again. Focus on the immediate tasks you have set for yourself each day, and praised yourself for each effort you have made--even if it was not successful. Try making a checklist so you get that moment of victory when you can cross something off.

Establish simple routines to help you, like sorting laundry into three hampers and laying out each day's clothes in advance. Take your plate to the sink and wash dishes as you cook so that at the end of dinner, when you are even tireder than usual because you are full, you won't have a mountain that you will have to keep until morning.

Find convenient and logical places to store things, and train yourself and your family to put things back when you are through using them. Get rid of things you and your family don't need.

On some low-energy days, it seemed like all you can accomplish is keeping things in their proper places. But that is an important part of housekeeping! And you should praise yourself for the effort you are making.

You will have to make changes, there is no doubt to that. You will have to work on keeping the expectations of yourself and your family realistic, delegating some tasks to others. Either within your family or professional help, establish routines that everyone follows, like picking up after yourself and encouraging others to do the same, pacing yourself, resting before you get tired, and praising yourself for the effort you are making.

All of these involve discipline applied a little at a time. You might even find that discipline is not an unwelcome burden, but rather a way of taking care of yourself. Start feeling better about yourself, your family, and your home. You should have to worry about people stopping by or the delivery man catching a glimpse of your dirty home. Get this taken care of sooner rather than later and save yourself a lot of stress.

Your Car

Driving safely and competently on the roads requires skills of high complexity and acute attention to the road and the traffic patterns. Sometimes, that just isn't possible. In the worst stages of CFS, most people will stop driving unless it is an emergency as they are simply too unwell to do so. The total energy output and muscular exertion required in driving and parking a car may trigger unpleasant symptoms such as painful muscles and exhaustion, or could make the person fall asleep while driving – which is deadly.

Helpful Hints

- Keep outside appointments to an absolute minimum, such as medical and other practitioner appointments only – if you can get them to come to your house, you might consider doing so.
- Ask a family member, or friend to drive you to important appointments or just to get you outside of the house.
- Red Cross has volunteer drivers who will provide transport to hospital appointments. You will probably need to negotiate a mutually suitable date and time with them, as they often arrange multiple pickups. They are very willing to work with you, however.
- Some local councils provide a community transport service for those who are sick or the elderly. This service provides transportation for people to attend social events and medical

appointments. You will need to register for this service prior to booking, and you may have to pay a small fee.

- Volunteer drivers are available in some areas funded under certain programs. Contact your insurance provider!
- The doctor's office or hospital may also provide community transport. Contact your local Service for information.
- For those who are severely ill, you need a doctor's referral to access non-essential ambulance transport to medical and hospital appointments.

When your condition has stabilized and you feel able to drive again, re-check the driving skills you will require for safe driving, such as:

- Coordination
- Parking
- Concentration
- Memory
- Energy
- Reaction time
- Judgment
- Precision
- Adequate eyesight
- Fair hearing
- Strength and muscle tone
- Information processing
- Defensive driving skills
- Updated knowledge of road rules

If you have not been driving for some time, it is advisable to refresh your driving skills prior to going out on the roads. This will highlight areas where you will need to lift your driving skills to a more competent level.

THINGS TO PRACTICE AND THINGS TO AVOID

There are several things that those living with CFS should do and those they must avoid in order to defeat the illness and live an abundant life without limitations.

Pace and Create a balance

Pacing is all about creating a balance between activities and taking rest. It is very easy to overwork one's self with too much exercise or activity. However, it is important to create a balance between the two. A patient must get to know when they are tired so they can stop and get enough sleep. In case they get tired during activities, they must stop and rest. It takes more time to recover from overworking one's self than it does to sleep regularly.

Do Not Compare Yourself to Others

The worst foul a CFS patient can commit is comparing themselves with others. Every person is unique; no two CFS patients are the same. It takes different therapies, medications, exercises and activities to treat different patients. This is the reason every patient is destined for different treatment program that suits them. In order to measure a patient's success or progress in treatment, only their past records can be used for comparison purposes.

Regular Visits to the Doctor

The patient should visit their physician regularly to ensure that their records are updated; the understanding and trust between them are also improved. The doctor should be experienced and knowledgeable in the treatment and management of chronic fatigue syndrome.

Maintain a Balanced Diet

Eat fresh fruits and vegetables, dark chocolates, sprouted pulses, and seeds, foods rich in iron and Vitamin B12, vegetable proteins, starchy foods and those high in fibers. Patients can also keep food diaries to help them track the foods they eat in order to ensure that they eat from all the food groups and determine those they are sensitive to and thus react to them. Caffeine, alcohol, and foods rich in sugars should be avoided at all times because they bring about energy bursts.

Avoid Stress

Although no proof exists of stress being the cause of the CFS, it is closely related to it and thus should be avoided at all cost. Setting achievable goals and keeping a flexible schedule can help reduce stress. Avoid news stories on televisions or opt for real life shows instead of watching television the whole time. Keep a personal journal, and don't discuss your help issues with other people. Anything that brings about anxiety should be entirely avoided as stressful events can bring about or cause this disorder.

Identify CFS Triggers

Patients should work closely with their doctors or physicians in order to determine the things that trigger worsening symptoms of CFS. Whether they are allergies, sensitivities, environmental or dietary in nature, understanding of the triggers defined helps patients to live a happy life without CFS.

Get Enough Rest

Getting adequate rest is essential for giving the body time to heal after an activity such as exercise. Avoid commitments and do not stress yourself trying to recall things that happened, in case the patient has problems with memory. Just relax and live life one step at a time.

Explore Alternative Therapies and medicine

Alternative medicine is said to work in the treatment of CFS. Patients should explore homeopathy, acupuncture, hypnotherapy and Reiki, among others. The combination of these in the exercise program of the patient should be tried out in order to find which method works best for their treatment process.

Share with Other CFS Patients

When patients with the same illness converge to discuss the problems they face, it gives them a sense of belonging and understanding that they are many of them suffering. This makes them more enthusiastic about themselves, the treatment program and generally, about living life with less or no limitations brought by CFS.

MANAGING STRESS – ENJOYING LIFE DESPITE CFS

When pressure of a mental or psychological nature overwhelms an individual, they are said to be stressed. Although the sensory system and the mind can be boosted through motivation and energy by minimal stress levels, it affects a person's physique and emotions negatively when in high levels. This is not suitable for a patient living with CFS. Since stress is an integral part of CFS, it is important to understand it. It can lead to anxiety and depression if not properly managed and treated. It can also trigger the symptoms of CFS and thus, worsening the patient's condition. Stress management is all about controlling and minimizing stress levels. There are various stress management techniques and methods that should be applied to patients in order to enjoy life without chronic fatigue syndrome. Let's take a look below at some therapy techniques and relaxation exercises for instant stress reduction.

Meditation

Meditation is a relaxation technique in which the mind is induced to a conscious state in order to make it calm and clear; it has a range of benefits like instant stress reduction. A 'mantra' word is said many times with eyes closed, either when performing an activity or while sitting; this is because there are various kinds of meditation. Some are performed when the body is still, and others require some form of body movement. Focusing on a single thought or thing is also used to quiet the mind during meditation. Inner self-awareness can result from meditation and its calming effects. The reflection of one's own life and profound thought, contemplation, are entailed in a meditation process.

Meditation has psychological and physical benefits because it heals the soul and the mind. Some of the physical benefits include a low heart rate during sleep, enhanced breathing rates, a younger-looking and supple skin, lower blood pressure and reduced stress hormone levels. Low-stress levels, improved concentration, mood and memory and reduced depression levels are some benefits the patient receives mentally when they meditate. When incorporated into the patient's lifestyle, meditation improves its quality and thus helping reduce the symptoms of CFS.

Deep Breathing

Shallow breathing and tension of the muscles can result from being stressed. Relaxed breathing allows for muscle relaxation and the evocation of hormonal stress. Deep breathing allows for full and deep lung cleanses. They should regularly be done, and they can instantly reduce stress because patients can take them anywhere at any time. However, quiet environments are recommended.

Deep Muscle Relaxation Techniques

Stress and tension can be relieved from tense body muscles through relaxation and stretching. The mind can also be relaxed through this technique that should last an average of 20 minutes.

Biofeedback

Stress can cause an abnormal level of certain functions of the body, such as breathing and heart rates, temperature, pressure and body muscle tension. Biofeedback allows for the measurement of these values regularly in order to monitor them. When an abnormal level is detected, the right action or measure is taken to rectify it in order to get it back to a normal level.

Other Techniques

Other techniques and ways of reducing and managing stress comprise of progressive muscle relaxation, body scan method of relaxation, mindfulness technique, visualization, yoga, Tai Chi, regular exercises, eating healthy foods, socialization and enjoying life. Have fun by living it to the fullest, enjoying a hobby, having a shower, seeking support and peace spiritually, enjoying laughter, living a healthy and active lifestyle and engaging in charity work. Cognitive behavioral therapy, listening to music that soothes the soul, use of art therapy, herbal home remedies including aromatherapy, fear assessment, time management, stress removal, massage, thinking positively, optimism, hypnosis and expression of love are all ways to cope with your condition.

STRONG QUOTES CONCERNING CFS

One of the biggest problems with suffering from CFS is that we feel like we are alone. It is something not many people talk about, so patients might not even know someone who is suffering from the disease. If you are feeling alone or lost, read these quotes and understand that you are never alone.

"Fatigue is what we experience, but it is what a match is to an atomic bomb."

—Laura Hillenbrand, author of Seabiscuit and Unbroken (NYT, "An Author Escapes From Chronic Fatigue Syndrome", February 4, 2011)

"The whole idea that you can take a disease like this and exercise your way to health is foolishness. It is insane."

—Dr. Paul Cheney, CFS researcher and clinician (comment made at the Invest in ME conference in May 2010)

"Don't tell me, "You don't look sick!" You don't look that insensitive either!"

—Anonymous

"Hopefully one day, my dream is that our medical community will produce a formal apology to the patients that—not having believed them all these years—they are facing a real illness."

—Dr. Jose Montoya, CFS researcher and clinician, Stanford University (during a lecture on Chronic Fatigue Syndrome at Stanford University on March 3, 2011)

"... a psychiatrist without compassion is a terrifying thing indeed."
—Dr. Deckoff-Jones in her July 31, 2011 blog post "Consensus" (directed at Prof. Wessely)

"The bad news is we don't know what causes it or how to treat it successfully. But the good news is that there are now over 4,000 published studies that show underlying biological abnormalities in patients with this illness. It's not an illness that people can just imagine that they have, and it's not a psychological illness. In my view, that debate, which has raged for 20 years, should now be over."
– Dr. Anthony Komaroff, CFS clinician, and researcher, Harvard Medical School (2006 Press Conference)

"... I'm not a chronic fatigue doctor, but I have learned a lot about chronic fatigue in the last six months and have spoken to a lot of patients. I'm absolutely convinced that when you define this disease by proper criteria, this is a very serious and significant medical disease, and not a psychological disease. It has the characteristics of a viral disease. It usually starts with a viral-like illness. If XMRV is not the causative agent — and it may well not be — there is still need by other groups to look for the next agent which may be the case."
– Dr. Harvey Alter, NIH Investigator (FDA Blood Products Advisory Committee meeting, 2010)

"...for those who have studied the disease for many years, it is apparent that the most serious issue in CFS is a kind of brain malfunction that may be caused by an infectious agent, or some other source that is, so far, poorly understood. But for most practitioners who can barely keep up with their schedules, it is vastly easier to dismiss an illness as imaginary than to grapple with brain physiology."
—Dr. David Bell, CFS clinician and researcher (Faces of CFS, ebook).

"Nearly every patient with CFS thinks of suicide at one time or another, but rarely can the impulse be blamed exclusively on mere physical pain and disability. I have discovered that most people learn to tolerate those things, particularly the tough breed of people who live out in the country. Instead, CFS sufferers are driven to suicide by loneliness and self-doubt, which arrive part and parcel with the disease itself. Although they are ill with a debilitating flu-like illness every day of their lives, neighbors and even friends and family insist they look "just fine." It's an unfortunate fact that our culture has yet to accept the harsh reality of chronic disease; often, its ravages are invisible to the naked eye. But CFS carries a terrible stigma, the burden of which weighs more heavily on them even than the burdens borne by most victims of chronic disease. The world seems to believe that people with CFS – a population the medical profession has yet to stamp with its imprimatur of "bona fide" – could "snap out of it" if they really wanted to. This utterly false perception of the disease is so widespread that, eventually, most patients with CFS, especially those who become increasingly isolated, have periods when they begin to suspect: 'maybe I am just crazy.'"

—Dr. David Bell, CFS clinician and researcher (Faces of CFS, ebook).

"We do not know the cause of CFS for the same reason that we do not know the cause of many neurologic diseases: we have not yet been clever enough to figure it out. If the word 'polarized' means that opinions will remain unchanged regardless of the evidence, I would like to think that this is not the case. And I am not sure that the CFS field is more polarized than other fields. The reception that the prion hypothesis (which states that a prion is a protein that can replicate without the use of nucleic acid) received for more than a decade comes to mind. So, too, does the current debate over the possible etiologic role of Epstein–Barr virus in multiple sclerosis.

—Dr. Anthony L. Komaroff, CFS clinician, Harvard Medical School

"CFS is controversial because the case definitions (that is, how the illness being studied is defined) of CFS consist exclusively of symptoms — and obviously anyone can say they have the constellation of symptoms that meets the case definition. Skeptics rightly ask whether there is evidence of objective biological abnormalities underlying CFS. In my judgment, the literature demonstrates many such abnormalities, both when patients with CFS are compared to healthy controls and when they are compared to patients with other fatiguing illnesses, such as multiple sclerosis or major depression. Many of the documented abnormalities involve the central and autonomic nervous systems. In my experience, most skeptics are unaware of the extensive literature citing such abnormalities and become less skeptical upon reading it."

—Dr. Anthony L. Komaroff, CFS clinician, Harvard Medical School

Question: "Some in the scientific community believe that immune findings are inconsistent and uncertain in ME / CFS. What is your comment on that?"

Answer: "I am so frustrated with those who say that, because we have been doing this for 25 years. Look at the studies of many patients – those who have a hundred or two hundred patients – and they tell you the same. It is not difficult. I mean immune findings in ME / CFS is proved. It is not controversial, and it is not just a hypothesis. There is immune activation, it is dysfunctional cells and a significant degree of malfunction of the immune system....I have no difficulty to say with great certainty that the immune

system in ME / CFS is not working as it should."
—Dr. Nancy Klimas, CFS researcher, and clinician, University of Miami

"The irony to me about that situation that we all chronically live in is the harder you try to protect the people around you from being uncomfortable with the fact that you are sick, the more invisible it becomes"
—Amberlin Wu, patient advocate (YouTube interview 2008)

Why, if I woke up, didn't I wake up?"
–John Herd, July 24, 2013

RESOURCES

Here are some quick resources from SolveCFS.org that you can check right now for help with Chronic Fatigue Syndrome, but please don't forget to grab the FREE list of resources provided as a Bonus Supplement to this book below!

http://solvecfs.org/mecfs-resources/patient-resources/
http://solvecfs.org/mecfs-resources/patient-resources/family-and-friends/
http://solvecfs.org/research/cfidsaa-research-program-for-researchers/
http://solvecfs.org/research/for-healthcare-providers/
http://solvecfs.org/mecfs-resources/patient-resources/solve-mecfs-initiative-2014-webinar-series/

Please visit our site online for more than 50 FREE Chronic Fatigue Syndrome resources all in one place!
http://www.plaid-enterprises.com/cfs

CONCLUSION

Research conducted over years to determine the root cause of CFS found results that conflict. Although some patients get well, in the long run, the condition and symptoms of others deteriorate with time. However, with medication, physical exercise, stress management, and treatment, there is hope for those living with this disorder. Moreover, no matter how long a patient suffers from CFS, they can be sure that it will never result in the failure of their body organs or even death.

It is not easy living with chronic fatigue syndrome, but despite its origin or cause being unknown, preventing and managing it is possible. Living an active and healthy lifestyle is a sure way of avoiding and managing this disorder. Patients living with CFS should not lose hope because they can live an abundant life without the limitations of this disorder. All it takes is living a more active life through regular exercise, engagement in physical activity and eating a balanced diet. Although the benefits of engaging in activities aimed at curbing this illness take time to be realized, patients must be optimistic, courageous, hopeful, persevering and positive thinking. There is no better way of living with chronic fatigue syndrome (without its limiting factors) than implementing the tactics discussed in this book. After all, it is time that will heal.

I personally want to thank you again for picking up this book! I sincerely hope the information contained will help you to understand the basics of Chronic Fatigue Syndrome, and more importantly, how to elevate your life past the limits of CFS. The next step is to put into practice the knowledge and employ the strategies we've discussed here to overcome these limitations and begin taking your life to the next level!

Finally, if you enjoyed this book, please take the time to share your thoughts and post a positive review on Amazon. I would greatly appreciate your support!

Thank you and good luck!

Kara Aimer

Please get your FREE Additional Bonus Resources for this Book HERE at:
http://www.plaid-enterprises.com/cfs

COPYRIGHT NOTICE

Printed in Great Britain
by Amazon